CORRECTION

Best Bust Arms and Ba

ISBN 0330 377418

The Publisher apologizes
To discover your resting metabolic rate, the figure you multiply
by should read 24, not 241.

And Finally . . .

This workout programme is challenging. It isn't difficult for your body, it's hard for your mind. Being determined to improve your body pays dividends you'll never regret because feeling good about yourself reaches deep into every area of you life. Being confident helps your career and your relationships. Feeling good about your body puts a smile on your face and cheers you up. In short, things seem to run more smoothly when you know you look good.

Stick with a healthy-eating plan and be strong. I can't pretend that it's always easy to steer clear of fattening foods: calorie-awareness is a burden until you get used to it but it will soon be second nature. Above all, think of the results. A good, enviable figure and the admiration of your circle last a lot longer than a slice of cake. Keep thinking about that as you do another set of Overhead Presses or Triceps Extensions! This plan will have good results in about six weeks and dramatic results after a few months. *No one was ever sorry they went for a walk. No one ever felt worse for a good stretch.* You're brilliant! Good luck!

MONICA GRENFELL is the *News of the World* Diet and Fitness Expert, read by millions. Her flat-stomach diet *Five Days to a Flatter Stomach*, her beauty diet plan *Fabulous in a Fortnight* and the sensational *Get Back Into Your Jeans Diet* (with its accompanying video) have all been runaway successes. All of Monica Grenfell's books are available from your local bookshop, or by sending a cheque or postal order as detailed below. Ask for details of her latest!

FABULOUS IN A FORTNIGHT
0 330 35368 3 £7.99 pb

5 DAYS TO A FLATTER STOMACH
0 7522 2130 2 £4.99 pb

THE GET BACK INTO YOUR JEANS DIET
0 330 37303 X £4.99 pb

MONICA'S FABULOUS BODY PLANS
Beautiful Bottom
0 330 37743 4 £2.99 pb
Best Bust, Arms and Back
0 330 37741 8 £2.99 pb
Fantastic Legs and Thighs
0 330 37740 X £2.99 pb
Marvellous Midriff
0 330 37742 6 £2.99 pb

Book Services By Post
PO Box 29
Douglas
Isle of Man IM99 1BQ

Credit card hotline 01624 675137.
Postage and packing free.

MONICA'S FABULOUS BODY PLANS

Best **Bust, Arms** AND **Back**

MONICA GRENFELL

PAN BOOKS

ADVICE TO THE READER

Before following any of the exercise or dietary advice
in this book it is recommended that you consult your
doctor if you suffer from any health problems or special
conditions or are in any doubt as to its suitability.

First published 2000 by Pan Books
an imprint of Macmillan Publishers Ltd
25 Eccleston Place, London SW1W 9NF
Oxford and Basingstoke
Associated companies throughout the world
www.macmillan.co.uk

ISBN 0 330 37741 8

9 8 7 6 5 4 3 2 1

A CIP catalogue record for this book is available
from the British Library.

Photography of Monica Grenfell by
Lesley Howling
Back cover photograph by Tony Ward,
direction by Lillie Gooch
Designed by Macmillan General Books
Design Department

Printed and bound in Belgium

Introduction

Everything about your upper body speaks volumes. A great bosom and back don't look just lovely – they're majestic. Pretty arms are classy. A good-looking pair of legs is lovely, but an eye-catching, creamy-skinned, feminine cleavage, arms and back are simply stunning. The old days of bra-burning, 'natural' busts and rounded shoulders are well and truly over, with firmness and voluptuousness taking centre stage again. You want to wear the fashions but does that mean practically setting up home in the gym or counting calories for ever? No, it doesn't. But if there's one word you must get into your head if you want to be successful in overcoming figure problems, it's 'consistency'. Routine, regularity and consistency are the keys to looking good. Yo-yo diet plans, on-off exercise routines and the attitude that counting calories is 'boring' – these are the reasons people have figure problems. Getting your bust, arms and back into fantastic shape is no worse than shopping or washing your hair or filling in your expenses form. OK, you'd rather someone else did it for you, but it's hardly laser surgery.

This book is all about how to achieve the upper body you've always wanted. We go mad for slim hips and a flat stomach and forget our top half. But go to a party in a glamorous evening dress and it isn't the state of your ankles everyone will be noticing. Yes, they all matter in the long run, but neglect your bust, arms and back and you'll regret it as you swelter in long sleeves and shapeless blouses. But don't worry. This book has all the solutions, especially if you simply don't know which exercise works best. For example, running won't help your arms. By getting a programme that is right for you, you can have firm, defined muscles, a taut back and a smooth cleavage.

Background

Your body was built for activity. Even though as cavewomen we wouldn't have spent our days hunting or chopping wood, we were designed for a range of activities rather greater than switching on the dishwasher. The muscles in our back enable us to make wide, sweeping movements similar to tennis-playing or window-cleaning, and our arms are capable of carrying heavy loads long distances. We've swapped hours of general domestic activity for a couple of hours half-heartedly pumping a pectoral machine. We get saggy boobs so decide to go for a run. This isn't the answer. But I'll give you three different workout options for that sensational upper body.

The bust is a slightly different matter when it comes to glamour because breasts have no muscles and breast tissue naturally shrinks with age. You can't exercise your breasts but you can tone your pectorals for a gorgeous cleavage. Arms and backs are also very simple because you use them every day anyway. This book is all about how to start, which exercises are best and how to keep it up. So what are you waiting for?

How It All Fits Together

Your 'starter kit' comes in the form of a tough skeleton, a lot of internal organs and a huge overcoat of muscles draped around the whole structure. The muscles cross joints and are fixed to a bone. Anything else you have on your body was put there by you, but the good news is that it's entirely in your hands as to how it all looks. Here therefore is the explanation of how to exercise.

Toning and sculpting

Traditional floorwork uses a high-rep overload, which means doing lots and lots of repetitions until the muscle you're working gets tired. You get the job done, but it takes ten times longer with ten times more effort.

Sculpting means exercising so you only need do a few reps per set – say sixteen. Both improve your tone but only sculpting can really change your shape. Sculpting uses much heavier weights for fewer repetitions – hence the term 'overload'.

What's 'overload'?

Overload sounds like serious bodybuilding but it's not. Overloading the muscle isn't dangerous and it isn't hard – it simply means *working a muscle to the point where changes have to happen* – and that means challenging a muscle to lift even heavier weights. Sometimes it is also called 'resistance'.

Resistance training

Resistance training is exactly what it sounds like. Imagine lifting your arm straight out in front of you – you have the weight of your arm as basic resistance – but now imagine someone pushing downwards on your arm to try to stop you lifting it. This is resistance! Any movement that uses an opposing force or a weight makes the job harder, and if your muscles work harder they need more calories, their fibres grow and your shape becomes more pronounced. Some everyday examples include sweeping, raking and vacuuming.

Stretching

Proper stretching makes the difference between a nice upper body and a sensational one. Stretching makes you stand tall: stretching stops your shoulders getting round as you hunch over your work, it improves the look of your arms and stops your neck becoming thick. Always stretch properly, and not just the usual, lacklustre stretching you might do at the end of an aerobics class. A few minutes isn't enough – always go for five to ten minutes a time.

Rules for stretching:
1 If you are not at the end of a training or workout session, warm up first by walking briskly or jogging on the spot, lightly.
2 Breathe slowly, deeply and evenly.
3 Do not stretch to the point where breathing becomes unnatural.
4 Do not overstretch.
5 Hold a stretch in a comfortable position – tension subsides as the stretch is held.

Your Questions Answered

My Bust Is Dreadful And Slack. It Used To Be Nice Until I Had Three Children And Now My Boobs Just Hang. I'm Only Twenty-Six And Worry That I'll Never Look Good Again. I Haven't Got A Weight Problem, In Fact I'm A Bit Thin. Any Hope For Me? Yes! Boobs can't be 'lifted' as such but as breasts are mostly fatty tissue with no muscles of their own, it's a case of having lost all your fatty 'support'. You need to gain muscle, and the pectorals, which are definitely there somewhere, need concentrated but sustained and consistent training for at least the next six months. The fibre will grow bigger every single week you're training, and they'll gradually plump out the skin on your chest.

When I Lift My Arms They Look Like Bats' Wings! The Fat Hanging Down Is Depressing Me. Will Exercise Do It Or Should I Diet? Although you probably DO need to lose some weight, the hanging flesh you can see is simply your muscle at rest. The triceps muscle runs down the back of your arm and only does its job when your arm is straightened. Do the triceps exercises religiously and follow the plan, and the slackness will soon disappear.

My Back Is Really Fat And I'm Simply Ashamed. My Skin Is Also Very Loose After Losing A Lot Of Weight Through Illness. How Can I Tighten Up My Skin And Get Rid Of All This Flab? You can't tighten skin, I'm afraid. However, don't be gloomy because the underlying muscles can be slightly increased in size, which won't make you look fat, just firm. This increase in size will 'plump out' your skin, as will a huge increase in the amount of water you drink.

I Don't See The Point In Exercising My Back When It's OK. It's My Boobs I'm Bothered About. Problems happen years before you see them. You don't eat a sweet and need a filling the next week. If your back isn't kept in good shape you'll know about it, and that's when people usually write to me and complain that 'suddenly' their back's gone all flabby! You absolutely mustn't neglect your back muscles, and they also balance your chest muscles. If you overtrain them and leave your back, you'll get classic bodybuilder's round shoulders, which are pulled inwards by the tight muscles.

I've Already Got Enormous Shoulders. How Can I Make Them Smaller? Aerobics, stretching and more stretching, and leave out the swimming and weight training.

Getting Motivated

It's not hard to get motivated to start off a fitness plan. Just look in the mirror! To lose three inches off your hips, lift your bottom and get a waist, you slog away night after night at the gym, lose an inch and a few pounds. The depression wears off. You've reached the 'plateau', where a bit of improvement's better than nothing. *But don't forget why you started.*

When you're 'too busy/stressed/harassed' for exercise . . .

1 Decide on a couple of days and times when you could exercise if push came to shove. Examples are when you're frittering time watching TV or generally fiddling about at home. I know that you've a lot of jobs to catch up on but you're probably spinning them out. Work faster!

2 Take trainers or easy shoes to work and do a twenty-minute walk in your lunch break to work up an appetite.

3 Make a decision to do one and then two tasks every week the 'old' way. Wash your car by hand, put the TV remote control in a drawer upstairs, clean all the windows. It's a start!

4 Do something! Everyone has an off-day, but don't give in and slump in a chair. Take the same time slot you reserved for your exercises and clear out a drawer, prune the roses, polish your shoes. You'll feel you've got something out of the day and your time won't have been wasted.

Losing Fat

Fat loss in the upper body is a tricky subject. You can't tell your body where to take its fat stores from, and you must avoid that dreadful 'toast-rack' effect on your chest. It's partly an inevitable sign of ageing unfortunately, but you CAN combat it by building muscle and not losing too much fat. They say that after forty, 'it's a woman's face or her figure' and I'd add to that 'and her cleavage'. However, things have changed a lot in modern times and women aren't ashamed to go and do weights to help improve their muscles. Don't make the mistake of thinking that everything you eat must be 'worked off'. Food isn't there to be worked off, it's there to keep you breathing and working and getting from A to B. If you do need to lose fat, only do so by the calorie-counting method.

How To Find Out How Many Calories You Need

Multiply your weight in pounds by 0.409. Multiply this number by 241 – this will give you your resting metabolic rate, in other words the minimum number of calories you need in a day.

Take in more calories than this – without significant extra exercise – and these are likely to be stored as fat. Always aim to use more than you eat.

So What Am I Going To Eat?

It isn't so much specific food but the nutrients in the food. The exercise programme in this book calls for a good amount of protein because you'll be training with weights, which means the muscles will be making new fibres and repairing themselves daily. Here are two of the most important nutrients:

Iron

Iron is important for all women, but in training you need extra iron to help the blood reach the working muscles. Lack of iron in your blood is evident if you feel breathless and exhausted after very little exercise or none at all, and of course tiredness. The best sources of iron are found in meat and other animal products. If you are a vegetarian I urge you to take a supplement, and also to eat nuts and dried fruits, remembering to count calories of course.

Carbohydrates

Carbohyrates are your energy source. You need long-term energy release found in starchy food like potatoes, rice and bread, and the fruit sugars from fruit and vegetables. Don't ever make the mistake of having a chocolate bar just before exercising to give you energy. It will do so, but after a short time you'll feel tired and listless again. Have a banana and some water, and refuel with carbohydrates AFTER exercising. You therefore should eat:

- Red meat
- Chicken
- Soya beans
- Yoghurt
- Sardines
- Almonds and brazil nuts
- Cheese

- Salmon
- Sunflower seeds
- Dried fruits especially apricots and figs
- Dark green vegetables
- All fruits

A balanced diet

A good diet would be:

Breakfast Grapefruit, home-made muesli with almonds and sunflower seeds, boiled egg and toast

Lunch Tuna fish salad, fruit salad

Main meal 6 oz fillet steak, jacket potato, salad or steamed broccoli and carrots, fromage frais with a fruit compote

When To Eat

Start strong . . . finish 'long'. Your FIRST meal of the day should be a 'dry' carbohydrate blast – you've been without food for about twelve hours so stoke up your supplies immediately with cereals, bread and other carbohydrate-filled foods. Your LAST meal of the day should be slow-release carbohydrates to stoke you up after training and see you through the night – hence the 'long' time they keep you hydrated and fuelled. You also need 'wet' carbohydrates to give you plenty of essential fluids to get those cells plumped-up – so make sure you eat fruit and vegetables in the evening. Try to avoid having your main meal of the day in the evening.

The 'Plateau'

Everybody reaches a 'plateau'. This is a sign of success because what you set out to achieve has been successful. Let me give you a good example – a daily one-hour brisk walk is excellent for your health, so if you were starting from nothing you would see a vast improvement quite quickly. Say you were a marathon-runner, though. If you had only an hour's brisk walk a day your body tone would actually get worse! *So whilst MAINTAINING a figure takes less effort than getting there, you must CHANGE the way you exercise to keep pace with your changing body shape.*

With diet, the same applies. Your body's getting used to being lighter and having less to carry around and this means the weight loss stops. Sticking to a diet of vegetables and lean meat at times like these can be soul-destroying but you must be positive. So remember:

1   Increase the EFFORT you put into exercise rather than the time spent, e.g. simply walk a lot faster so you do 2 miles instead of 1½ miles in thirty minutes.
2   Increase the weight you're using to challenge your muscles.
3   Increase the number of sets.
4   Vary your diet by introducing food you've never tried before.
5   DON'T try to speed up weight loss by cutting calories even further. Stick to your three meals a day, increase your exercise and the pounds will soon start to drop again.

Now turn the page for your step-by-step exercise plan.

The Exercises

WHAT YOU NEED You will need free weights for most of these exercises. I suggest two sets of 1lb wristband weights, plus 3lb and 5lb hand weights. Don't think you can get away with bottles of water or tins of beans either – they are not made for gripping and you need the proper, professional equipment if you want to succeed. **NOTE** As any upper body workout uses weights, you must observe correct form – otherwise you could do yourself a bad injury:

1 Make a point of getting into the correct starting position.
2 Breathe correctly – in as you line up to make the move and out as you either lift, pull, push or generally make the effort.
3 Don't use momentum by swinging your weights – this makes the move easier for your muscles and you won't get the results you're after.
4 Remember your 'helping' muscles – your abdomen and back muscles play an important part in stabilizing your body during most exercise, so take a second to pull in, lift up and provide that 'cage' of strength and stability.

Your Muscle Structure

The muscles in the upper body are complex, and made to perform a range of movements. Like all muscles they were designed for strength, flexibility and power, but don't let that put you off – you are going to tone them for firmness and beauty!

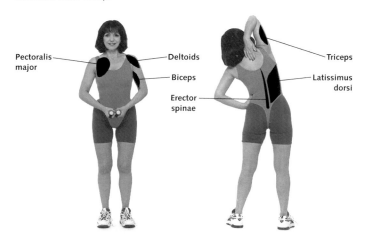

Pectoralis major

Deltoids

Biceps

Erector spinae

Triceps

Latissimus dorsi

The triceps

The triceps is a large fleshy muscle with three heads (the triceps brachii, situated at the back of your arm, originates in the shoulder blade and attaches to the elbow with a single tendon). The action of the triceps is to straighten your arm.

Triceps Extension

1 Stand sideways to a chair and place one knee on it, holding the chair for support.

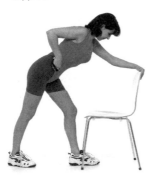 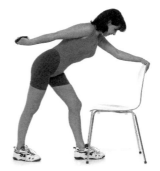

2 In the other hand hold a 3lb weight at your waist, elbow raised. Keep your elbow close to your back, don't let it drift out to the side. Breathe in and tighten your abdominal muscles.

3 Slowly straighten your arm, making sure you don't 'lock out' your elbow. Feel the back of your arm tightening and make sure the grip on your weight is light (or you'll be straining your forearm). Release and repeat. Do twelve, change arms and repeat. A set is twelve each side.

Triceps Stretch

Stretch the triceps by lifting each arm in turn and reaching down between your shoulder blades. Support the arm with the other hand. Hold for twenty seconds.

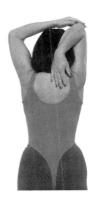

The biceps

The biceps muscles (biceps brachii) oppose the triceps, so you should always exercise them at the same time for perfect body balance. Don't ignore your biceps as a 'man's thing' because flabby biceps can look like fatty arms! The purpose of the biceps is to move the lower arm closer to the upper arm by bending the elbow.

Hammer Curl

1 Stand with feet slightly apart, holding weights. Bend your knees slightly, keep your palms turned inwards and your elbows close to your body.
2 One at a time, curl each weight up towards your upper arm, stopping short of the elbow, being in a fully-bent position. (This takes the effort out of the move.)
3 Lower slowly, again being sure not to let your elbows straighten and alternate arms. Do twenty-four, rest and repeat. A set is twenty-four.

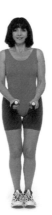
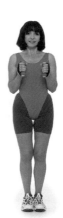

Supinated Bicep Curl

This exercise is exactly the same as the Hammer Curl, but this time you turn the palms upwards each time you make the move. Return to palms inwards as you lower. A set is twenty-four.

One-arm Wall Stretch

1 Stand sideways to a wall and place one hand on it, palms flat and elbow slightly bent, the hand level with your shoulder.

2 Slightly turn your body outwards, away from the wall. Feel the stretch in your shoulder and front of your arm. Do one stretch each side, stretch, then do two sets of Triceps Extensions, stretch.

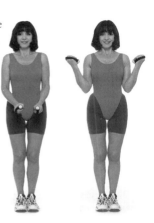

The deltoids

The main shoulder muscle is the deltoid. It is one large, flat triangular muscle that gives the shoulder its round look. The action of the deltoid is to take the arm away from the body, and to rotate the shoulder both inwards and backwards.There are three heads to the deltoid, so it takes three movements to work it.

Front-Delt Raises

1   Using 3–5lb weights stand with feet comfortably apart, abdomen pulled in and knees slightly bent. Lengthen your neck and lower your shoulders. Breathe in.
2   Breathe out as you raise one weight at a time, starting with the palms inwards but twisting so your elbow faces the floor and your palm faces upwards and slightly out to the side. Keep your elbows slightly bent. Alternate arms. Do twelve each side, rest and repeat. A set is twenty-four, twelve each arm.

Middle-Delt Raises

1 Stand with your feet close together, knees nearly touching and slightly bent. Pull in your abdominals and bend forwards slightly. Grip your weights in a palms-facing position as shown in the picture. Breathe in.

2 Breathe out as you lift the weights to the sides, keeping your elbows slightly bent. Don't raise your hands higher than your elbows. Do twelve slowly, rest and repeat. A set is twelve.

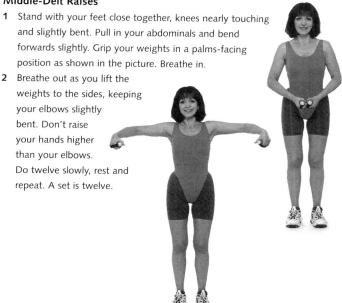

Rear-Delt Raises

1 Stand with feet together, abdominal muscles pulled tightly for stability, knees slightly bent, lean forwards. Holding 3lb weights as shown, palms facing inwards, breathe in.

2 Breathe out and raise one weight out and slightly behind you. It is difficult to raise your arm very high. Do twelve with one arm then change sides. A set is twelve each arm.

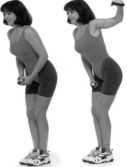

Shoulder Stretch

To stretch your shoulders, place your palms on your buttocks, fingers pointing directly downwards. Rotate your shoulders backwards. Now press your elbows close together as if you were trying to get them to meet (they won't). Keeping your elbows back and hands in place, press your shoulders forwards as far as you are able.

Push-backs

This is a combination exercise for triceps and rear deltoids.

1 Holding weights suitable for your level, stand with feet together. Bend your knees and tighten your abdominals for support. Hold your weights in front of you as shown, elbows slightly bent. Breathe in.

2 Breathe out as you sweep the weights backwards and outwards so they end up behind you and your shoulder blades are squeezing together. Your hands might touch, but don't worry if you need to work up to this. This is the peak of the contraction so hold the position for three seconds before releasing. Sweep back to the front again and repeat very slowly and deliberately. Do ten, rest and repeat. A set is ten.

**Make sure your neck stays long and doesn't arch.
Keep your shoulders pressed back and down.**

'Scoops'

This is a combination exercise for biceps and front deltoids.

1 Holding one weight and with your other hand resting on your thigh, knees bent, lean slightly forwards and hold abdominals in tightly. Turn your palm upwards, elbow facing the floor.

2 Breathe out, raising the weight straight up in a 'scooping' movement, hand level with your shoulders. Hold for a count of five, release. Do sixteen, rest and change hands. A set is sixteen each side.

Overhead Press

This exercise targets the triceps, shoulders and upper back.

1 Using your heavier weights, stand with
   your knees slightly bent and
   abdominal muscles pulled in.
   Breathe in.
2 Breathe out as you raise the
   weights directly overhead.
   Twist your hands as you do this, so
   your palms face each other at the
   top of the move. Lower and repeat.
   Do sixteen, rest and repeat. A set
   is sixteen.

Tip When you come to a 'rest'
between sets, pause for about ten
to twenty seconds, no longer. You
need to keep up the momentum in
your muscles and not allow them to
become cold.

The back

The main muscles in your back are the latissimus dorsi, trapezius, infra-spinatus and teres major, plus of course your spinal erectors, which stabilize you through all the exercises for both upper and lower body.

Latissimus Dorsi This is a huge sheet of muscle that starts as a large expanse across the back and 'fastens' into your humerus, the long bone that runs through your upper arm. Slack 'lats' are responsible for the rather unattractive bulge that shows under our bras.

Trapezius This is a big flat, triangular muscle that starts in the base of your skull and inserts into your shoulder blades and collarbone. Known as 'traps', when it is overdeveloped as in bodybuilding it is responsible for that 'bull-necked' appearance. Don't worry though – nicely toned traps pull your shoulders back and encourage beautiful posture.

One-arm Rows (1st position)

1 Stand with one knee on a chair, abdominal muscles pulled well in and back straight. Hold one of your heavier weights in one hand. Breathe in.
2 Breathe out as you raise the weight so it is close to your waist. Your elbow is still close to your body, not out to the side. You should feel your shoulder muscles pushing closer together.
3 Release the weight slowly to the starting position, inhaling as you do so.

You should feel your shoulder blades moving
further apart as your muscle 'pays out' your arm
to the floor. Do ten. Change arms and repeat.
A set is ten each side.

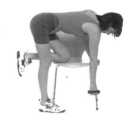

One-arm Rows (2nd position)

1 Start as for previous exercise.
2 This time as you raise the weight, lift your
  elbow out to the side. This slightly changes the
  angle and exercises a different part of your back.
  Do ten. Change arms and repeat. A set is ten
  each side.

The best exercise for the back is swimming,
especially the breaststroke, as the water provides
maximum resistance. Other exercises need gym equipment:

- The 'lat pulldown' – using both wide and narrow grip
- Rowing machine – try to use slow, intense movements and warm up first.

Lat Stretch-out

Stand upright and raise your right arm. Place it behind your head with a bent elbow. Take hold of your elbow with your left hand and gently press it towards your head. Feel the stretch in your back, below the armpit. Now bend over to the left as far as you can go, feeling the stretch in your side and back. Hold for a count of twenty. Change arms and repeat.

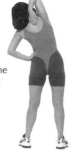

The bust and chest

The chest area uses several muscles to keep it 'plumped-up' with healthy muscle – and to avoid that 'toast-rack' look!

Pectoralis Major and Minor

The large, fan-shaped pectoral muscle covers the chest and also forms part of the armpit. Its action is to draw your arm forwards and across your chest and is used in a 'hugging' movement, or any move that involves pulling upwards, such as in climbing. The pectoralis minor lies beneath the larger muscle and comes into play when lowering your shoulder.

Press-ups

This combination exercise is easy to do, requires no equipment and works the shoulders, triceps and chest.

1   Take position on your hands and knees, with your feet raised off the floor and crossed. Your hands should be about shoulder-width apart. Breathe in and tighten your stomach muscles.

2   Slowly lower yourself, taking care not to let your stomach or back dip (remember that 'cage of strength' supporting your mid-section). Breathe out as you do so.

3   Raise up again, making sure you don't lock-out your elbows, which would take the effort away from the working 'prime mover' muscles. Repeat the press-up ten times. A set is ten. Have a short break of about thirty seconds, repeat another set.

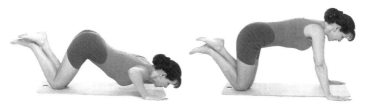

Ball Squeeze
You need a large beach ball or football for this exercise.

1 Stand tall, with stomach pulled in tightly, chest lifted. Hold the
   ball between your forearms as in the picture. Breathe in.
2 Breathe out as you start slow, rhythmic squeezes of the ball
   between your elbows. You should feel your upper chest muscles
   tightening with each squeeze. Do ten slowly, then twenty double
   time and another ten slowly. This is a set.

'Flyes'

1 Lie on the floor, knees bent. Holding your heavier weights, extend your
   arms to the sides at ear level, palms up. Breathe in and press your spine
   downwards so you feel the floor in the small of your back.
2 Breathe out as you lift the weights, turning your hands so your little
   fingers face one another. Return the weights to their starting position
   and repeat. Do a set of twelve slowly, rest then repeat.

Arching Stretch

This is just one simple all-round chest and shoulder stretch.

Take position on the floor, your hands flat behind you, fingers facing away from your body. Arch your back but not your neck. Press your ribcage upwards and out. Hold for thirty seconds. Release and repeat, trying to increase the stretch by taking your fingertips further away from your body. If you are new to exercise, stretch gently.

Back Strengthener

This exercise is vital to balance out your body after exercise, toning and strengthening all the muscles of the middle and lower back, plus shoulders.

1 Lie as shown, face down, fingers interlaced loosely behind your back. Keep your legs together. Breathe in.
2 Breathe out as your lift both legs and chest. Do not arch your neck. Hold for about six seconds, release and breathe in again. Repeat six times. This is a set.

Exercises for All-round Fitness

A truly Fabulous Body means all of it – not just the bit you don't like! If you work one part to the exclusion of others you could risk injury from lack of muscle balance. Try to insert daily abdominal and back strengthening exercises, and always stretch out leg muscles after running, using a treadmill, bike or stepper. Here are two stretches for your legs and one exercise for your midriff to help your all-round plan.

Calf Stretch Against a Wall
Stretch calves and thighs with this simple exercise.

Lean with both palms flat against a wall. Place your right foot 6in from the wall and take a step backwards with your left foot. Allow your heel to press flat to the floor. Hold the stretch for twenty seconds. Now just inch your foot backwards again a few centimetres and hold again. Change feet and repeat.

Standard Gluteal Stretch

Don't forget to stretch out buttock muscles with this easy stretch.

Lie on your back. Straighten one leg while bringing the other knee in towards your chest as far as you can. Do not let your lower leg bend off the floor. Hold for thirty seconds. Change legs and repeat.

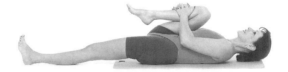

The Midriff Curl

Always finish your workout with abdominal strengthening exercises like this one.

1 Lie flat on the floor with your knees bent. Place your palms on your thighs and breathe in.

2 Breathe out as you slowly curl your neck slightly and press your spine downwards. Curl up just a few inches. Let your palms slide towards your knees. Your neck should be relaxed. Blow out rhythmically then release to the floor. You should be able to do no more than six a minute. A set is six.

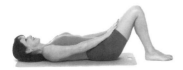
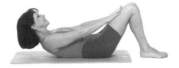

Fitness Walking

Although the three plans I have devised for you concentrate on home or gym exercise, you must always include walking in your life. But not any old walking! Fitness walking is brisk and purposeful, and observes good physical form. It improves circulation, loads your bones for strength, burns more calories long-term than short 'blasts' of exercise, and the daylight and fresh air help release endorphins – the feel-good hormones responsible for keeping low moods away.

Try to time your steps per minute (s.p.m.) before you get going, so you have an idea what 140 s.p.m. feels like. This exercise can also be done using a treadmill.

1 Always warm-up with three minutes at about 2½ m.p.h., this is about 90 steps per minute (s.p.m.).
2 Progress to 3½ m.p.h. (120 s.p.m.).
3 Aim for 4–4½ m.p.h. (140–160 s.p.m.).
4 Lean very slightly forwards, feeling your waist 'lifting' out of your waistband. Tighten your tummy muscles and feel as if you are leaning into a very strong gale.
5 Close fists lightly and pump your arms as you walk.
6 Lengthen your neck, feeling your spine in one straight line. Relax your shoulders.
7 Keep your feet hip-width apart. Concentrate on tightening your buttocks with each step. Try to think about each stride.
8 Strike the ground with each heel purposefully. Try to take long strides, feeling as if you are 'pulling back' the ground with each step.

Good! This is fitness walking, to improve your overall shape enormously.

Putting It All Together

You'll now be keen to put your new motivation into action, so to help you, I have devised three plans. You can chop and change between the plans, or devise your own.

Plan 1. The Quick-Fix, Any Time Home Plan

This plan takes just eighteen to twenty minutes and incorporates stair climbing, stair running, stair stepping, floorwork and stretches. Unlike the other two plans, which progress over four weeks, this is the same plan to fix in your mind for good, so eventually you won't need to keep referring to your book.

What you need A flight of stairs, ankle weights (optional)

When to do it While your supper's cooking, while the children are bathing, first thing Sunday morning, when it's wet outside, that irritating gap in the evening's TV viewing!

Stair walking and running Change into loose clothing or full leotard and leggings (this might make you feel more businesslike) and be sure to wear trainers. Walk up and down your stairs. Stair running is as it sounds. Keep up the momentum! *Sets of stair walking mean up and down once, twice and so on.*

Monday

STAIR EXERCISES:

Two sets of walking, two sets of
    running, two sets of walking

FLOORWORK:

One set of Hammer Curls (p.20)
    with 1–3lb weights

One set of Supinated Bicep Curls
    (p.21) with 1–3lb weights

One set of Front-Delt Raises (p.22)
    with 1–5lb weights

One set of Middle-Delt Raises (p.23)
    with 3lb weights

One set of Rear-Delt Raises (p.24)
    with 3lb weights

Repeat last three exercises

One set of Triceps Extensions (p.18)

One set of Scoops (p.26)

One set of Push-backs (p.25)

One set of Overhead Presses (p.27)

Repeat last three exercises

Two sets of Midriff Curls (p.36)

Shoulder Stretch (p.24)

Tuesday

Thirty-minute fitness walk (120–140
    s.p.m.)

FLOORWORK:

One set of One-arm Rows
    (pp.28–29) in both positions

One set of Ball Squeezes (p.32)

Two sets of 'Flyes' (p.32)

Repeat Ball Squeezes (p.32)

One set of Press-ups (p.31)

Two sets of 'Flyes' (p.32)

Repeat last two exercises

Two sets of Midriff Curls (p.36)

Arching Stretch (p.33)

Wednesday

Rest, but have a fitness walk

Thursday
As Monday

Friday
As Tuesday

Saturday or Sunday
STAIR EXERCISES:
Three sets of walking, step on and
    off bottom stair 100 times,

change leg after twenty
100 skips
Repeat Monday, Triceps Extensions
to Midriff Curls
Repeat Tuesday, second Ball
Squeezes to Midriff Curls
Two sets of Midriff Curls

Time for the week: four hours thirty
minutes

Plan 2. Gym Routine

Equipment Exercise bike or stepper, rowing machine, lat pulldown machine,
pec/dec machine, 3–5lb weights, treadmill, bar (weight to suit)

Monday
Five-minute warm-up on exercise
    bike or stepper
Ten minutes rowing
FLOORWORK:

Calf Stretch Against a Wall (p.34)
Triceps Stretch (p.19)
Shoulder Stretch (p.24)
2 x 12 lat pulldown, 2 x 10 pectoral
    squeezes, repeat

FLOORWORK:

One set of Press-ups (p.31)

One set of Push-backs (p.25) with
    3lb weights

Two sets of One-arm Rows (p.29)
    with 3–5lb weights*

Two sets of 'Flyes' (p.32) with 3–5lb
    weights*

Shoulder Stretch (p.24)

Time: thirty minutes

*   Start with 1lb wrist weights if
    you are a beginner

Tuesday

Treadmill: five minutes warm-up at 3
    m.p.h., twenty minutes at 4.3
    m.p.h., five minutes cool down
    at 3 m.p.h.

Calf Stretch Against a Wall (p.34)

Get your 1–3lb weights

FLOORWORK:

One set of Front-Delt Raises (p.22)

One set of Middle-Delt Raises (p.23)

One set of Rear-Delt Raises (p.24)

Repeat with 2–5lb weights

Change to 3lb weights

One set of Triceps Extensions (p.18)

One set of Hammer Curls (p.20)

One set of Supinated Bicep Curls (p.21)

Add 1lb wrist weights and repeat

Change to a bar

One set of Scoops (p.26)

Now use 3–5lb weights

One set of Overhead Presses (p.27)

Repeat last two exercises

Triceps Stretch (p.19)

Shoulder Stretch (p.24)

Lat Stretch-out (p.30)

Arching Stretch (p.33)

Ten minutes on bicycle

Four sets of Midriff Curls (p.36)

Back Strengthener (p.33)

Calf Stretch Against a Wall (p.34)
Standard Gluteal Stretch (p.35)
One set of Midriff Curls (p.36)
Time: one hour

Wednesday
Rest, but have a fitness walk

Thursday
Five-minute warm-up on the
    exercise bike
Fifteen minutes strong rowing
FLOORWORK:
Repeat Monday, Calf Stretch to
    One-arm Rows
Four sets of Midriff Curls (p.36)
Fifteen-minute strong swim
Time: fifty-five minutes

Friday
Five minutes on treadmill at 3 m.p.h.
Twenty-five minutes on stepper:
twenty minutes walking, five
    minutes cool down
Ten minutes strong rowing
FLOORWORK:
Repeat Tuesday, Front-Delt Raises
    to Arching Stretch with weights
    increasesd by 1lb
Triceps Stretch (p.19)
Time: forty-five minutes

Saturday
Complete rest

Sunday
Thirty-minute strong swim
Five sets of Midriff Curls (p.36)
Triceps Stretch (p.19)
Time: forty-five minutes

Total time for the week:
approximately four hours plus
fitness walks

 MONICA'S FABULOUS BODY PLAN

In the second and subsequent weeks increase weights gradually if you want to build muscle. Keep weights constant but increase the number of light repetitions to maintain tone but decrease size.

Plan 3. Combination Workout Using Cycling, Swimming And Home Exercise

Before beginning Week 3 remember what I said about overload (p.6). Think about increasing your weights by 1–2lbs this week.

	Week 1	Week 2	Week 3	Week 4
Monday	(Cycling)	(Cycling)	(Cycling)	(Cycling)
	5-min warm-up	5-min warm-up	5-min warm-up	5-min warm-up
	10 mins higher gear	10 mins higher gear	10 mins higher gear	10 mins higher gear
	10 mins hill climb	15 mins hill climb	20 mins hill climb	20 mins hill climb
	5 mins cool down	5 mins cool down	5 mins cool down	5 mins cool down

	Standard Gluteal Stretch	Standard Gluteal Stretch	Standard Gluteal Stretch	Standard Gluteal Stretch
	Calf Stretch Against a Wall	Calf Stretch Against a Wall	Calf Stretch Against a Wall	Calf Stretch Against a Wall
	2 x 12 Triceps Extensions	2 x 12 Triceps Extensions	2 x 12 Triceps Extensions	4 x 12 Triceps Extensions
	24 Hammer Curls	24 Hammer Curls	24 Hammer Curls	24 Hammer Curls
	2 x 16 Scoops	2 x 16 Scoops	4 x 16 Scoops	4 x 16 Scoops
	3 x 6 Midriff Curls	16 Overhead Presses	16 Overhead Presses	16 Overhead Presses
	Repeat stretches	24 Front-Delt Raises	24 Front-Delt Raises	24 Front-Delt Raises
	6 Midriff Curls	2 x 12 Flyes	2 x 12 Flyes	2 x 12 Flyes
	10 Press-ups	2 x 10 Press-ups	2 x 10 Press-ups	2 x 10 Press-ups
		3 x 6 Midriff Curls	3 x 6 Midriff Curls	3 x 6 Midriff Curls
		Repeat Stretches	Repeat Stretches	Repeat Stretches
		6 Midriff Curls	6 Midriff Curls	6 Midriff Curls
Time	50 mins	55 mins	1 hour	1 hour 5 mins

Tuesday	30-min swim	30-min swim	30-min swim	40-min swim
	All Stretches	All Stretches	All Stretches	All Stretches
Time	**35 mins**	**35 mins**	**35 mins**	**40 mins**

Wednesday	Complete rest	Complete rest	Complete rest	Complete rest

Thursday	45-min cycle	45-min cycle	40-rowing	10-min cycle
	10 mins rowing	10 mins rowing	10 mins cycling	45 mins rowing or swimming
	100 skips	100 skips	100 skips	100 skips
	2 x 12 Front-Delt Raises	2 x 12 Front-Delt Raises	2 x 12 Front-Delt Raises	4 x 12 Front-Delt Raises
	2 x 12 Middle-Delt Raises	2 x 12 Middle-Delt Raises	2 x 12 Middle-Delt Raises	4 x 12 Middle-Delt Raises
	3 x 10 Press-ups	3 x 10 Press-ups	4 x 10 Press-ups	4 x 10 Press-ups
	Standard Gluteal Stretch	Standard Gluteal Stretch	Standard Gluteal Stretch	Standard Gluteal Stretch
	Calf Stretch Against a Wall	Calf Stretch Against a Wall	Calf Stretch Against a Wall	Calf Stretch Against a Wall
	6 Midriff Curls	6 Midriff Curls	6 Midriff Curls	6 Midriff Curls
	5 x 6 Midriff Curls	5 x 6 Midriff Curls	5 x 6 Midriff Curls	5 x 6 Midriff Curls
Time	**1 hour**	**1 hour**	**1 hour 15 mins**	**1 hour 15 mins**

Friday	45-min walk	45-min walk	45-min walk	45-min walk
	Yoga class*	Yoga class*	Yoga class*	Yoga class*
Time	45 mins	45 mins	45 mins	45 mins

Saturday	As Monday	As Monday	As Monday	As Monday

Sunday	Complete rest	Complete rest	Complete rest	Complete rest
Total time for the week	4 hours	4 hours 10 mins	4 hours 35 mins	4 hours 50 mins

* Try to fit in a yoga or Pilates class once or twice a week if possible for the ultimate in beautiful bust, arms and back.